Introducti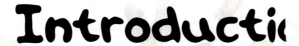

My goal is to demystify herbalism, making it simple and enjoyable to understand. To this end, I have written a children's book about herbs to ignite interest in young minds and simplify the subject for adults, ensuring it is both enjoyable and memorable.

I aim to inspire both children and adults to delve into herbalism, whether for professional purposes or home use. I hope you find joy in this book and feel compelled to share it with friends and family. Such a simple act could kindle the herbalist within, potentially benefiting many in the future.

- Mourab Raw Maraby

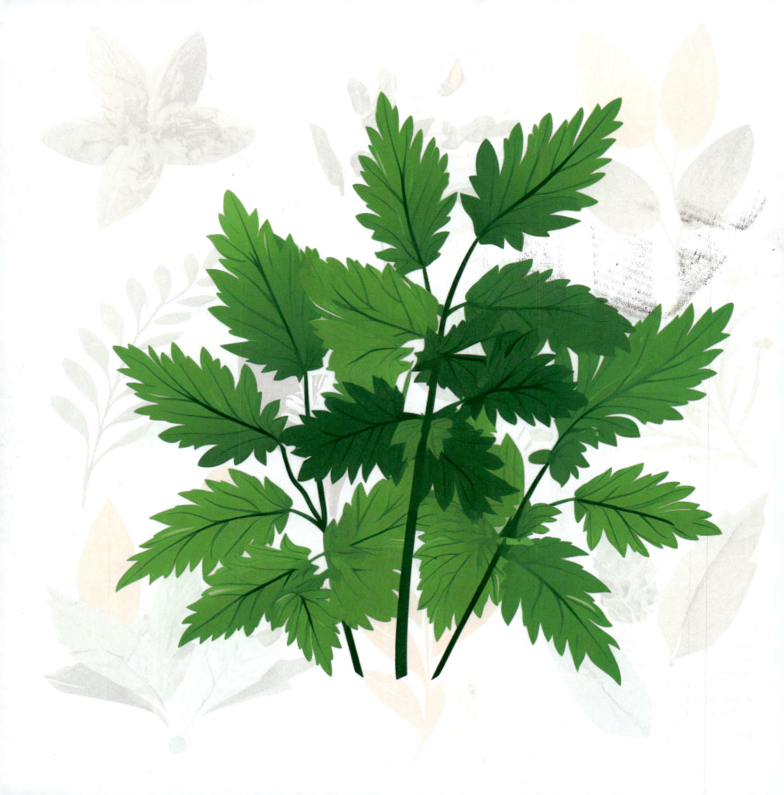

Once upon a time in a charming village, there lived a young girl named Lily. She had a secret talent that made her very special — she was an herbalist! Lily knew all about the magical powers of plants and herbs, but her favorite was the humble Nettle.

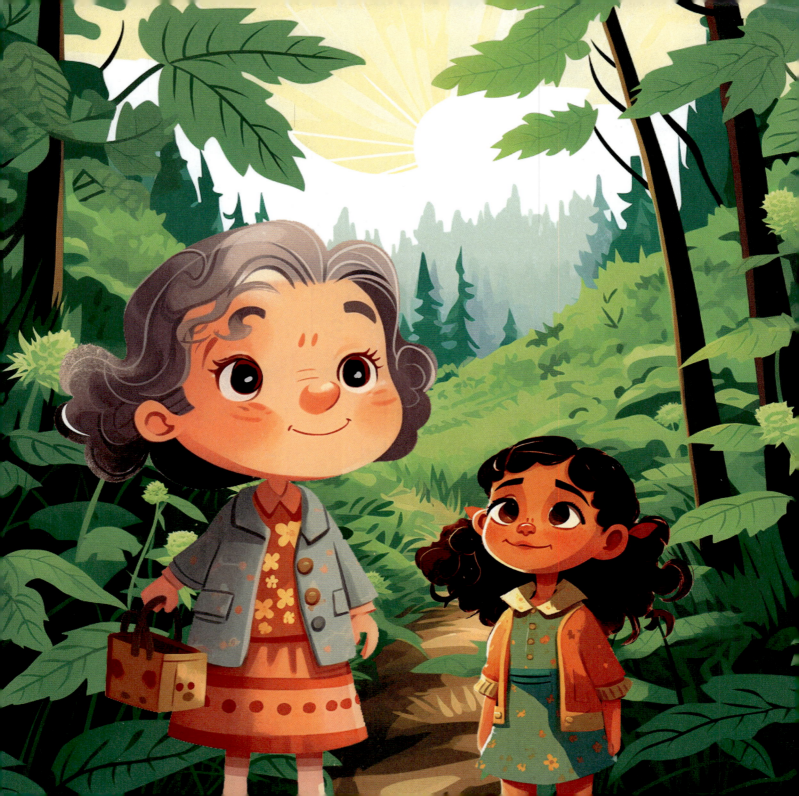

One sunny morning, as Lily was exploring the forest, she met her friend, Grandma Rose, who had a kidney problem. Grandma Rose looked tired and unwell. Lily knew just what to do.

Lily brewed a warm cup of nettle leaf tea and gave it to Grandma Rose. She explained how nettle leaf could help with kidney problems. The tea helped cleanse Grandma Rose's blood, and over time, her kidneys started feeling better. She didn't need dialysis anymore, and her smile returned!

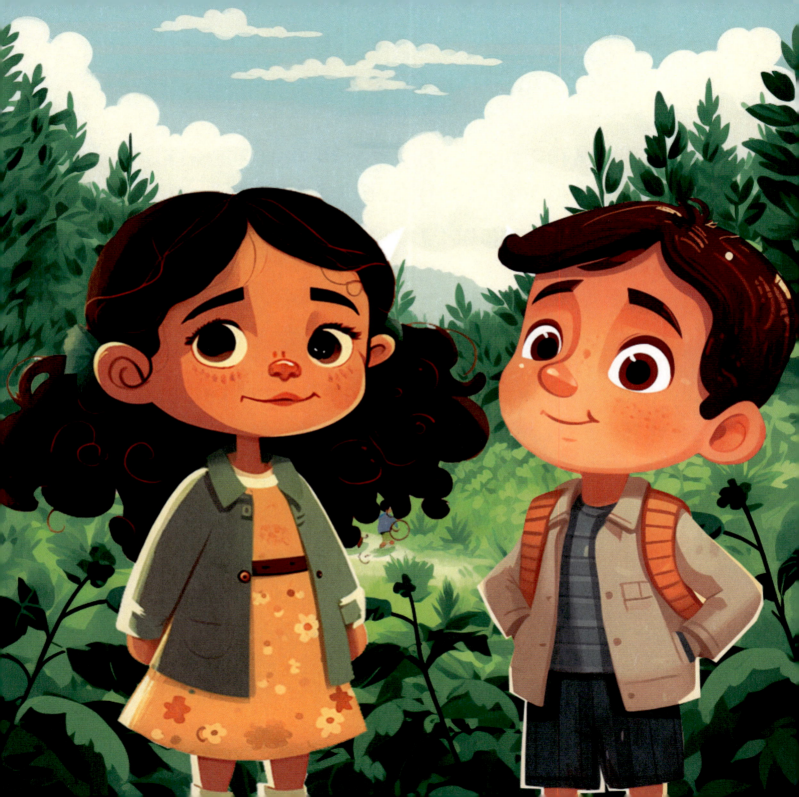

As Lily continued her adventures, she stumbled upon a stinging plant — the nettle. She carefully picked its leaves, which had tiny hairs that could sting if touched. Lily knew that these leaves were like hidden treasures for herbalists.

One day, Lily met her friend Timmy, who had terrible allergies. He sneezed and sniffled all day long. Lily made Timmy a special nettle leaf tea. It had a magical way of calming his allergies and helped him breathe better. No more sneezing fits for Timmy!

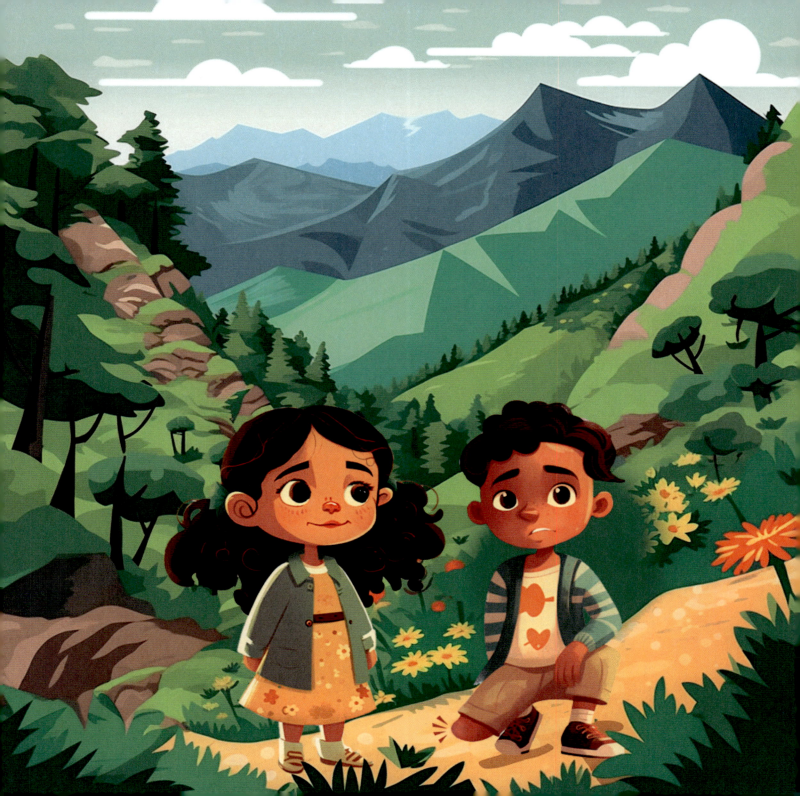

Lily's adventures took her deep into the forest, where she met Lucas, a brave explorer. Lucas had been hiking for days and had sore joints and aching muscles. Lily brewed him a soothing nettle leaf tea. The tea's power reduced Lucas's pain and helped him keep exploring the forest.

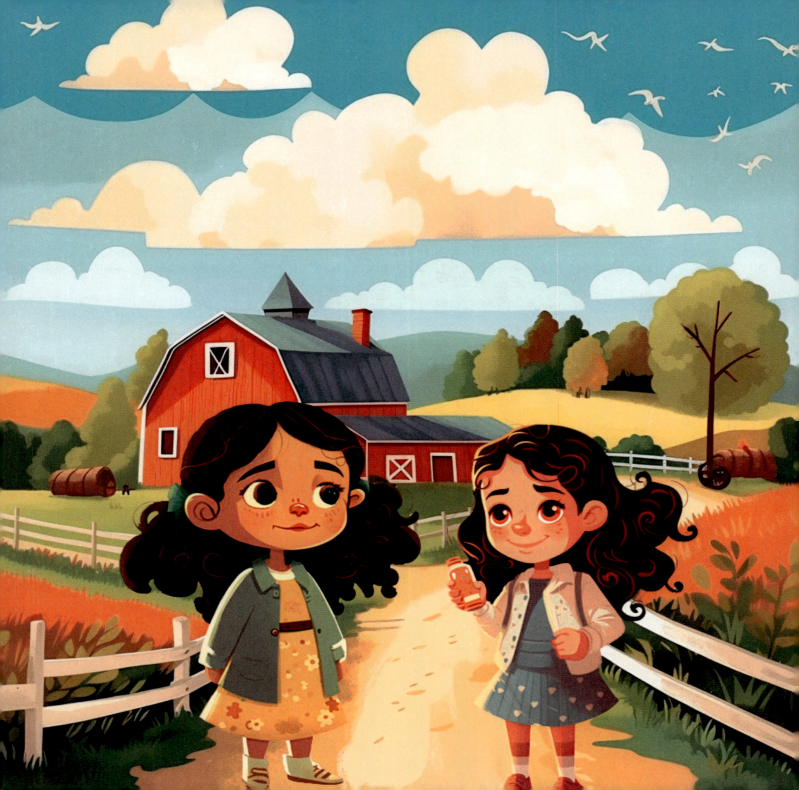

One cloudy afternoon, Lily met Mia, who felt tired all the time because she had anemia. Lily knew that nettle was rich in iron, just what Mia needed. She made a special nettle leaf tonic for Mia, and soon she had more energy, and her rosy cheeks returned.

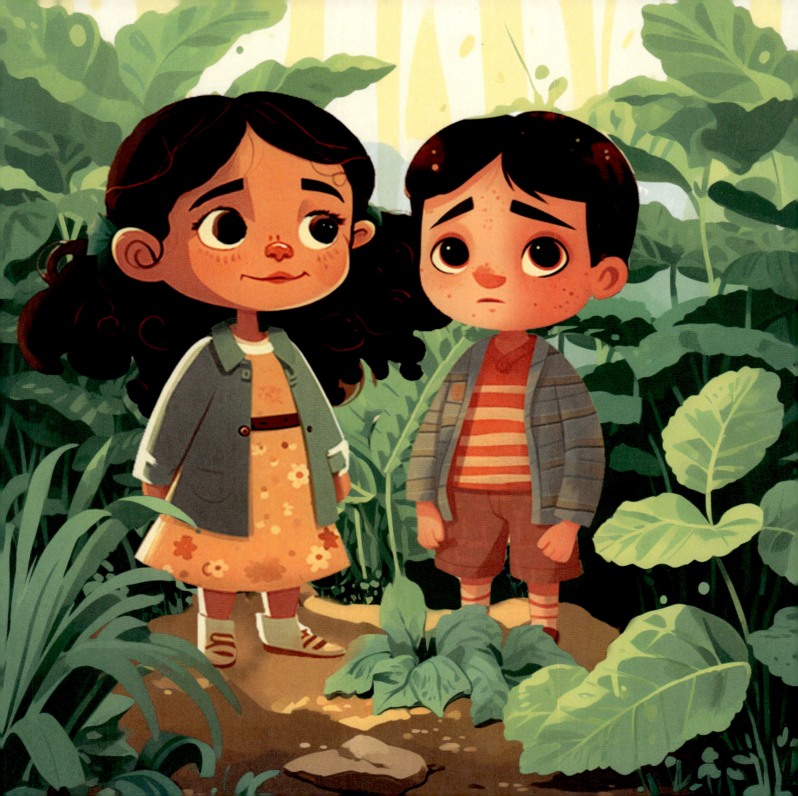

Lily's adventures continued, and she discovered that nettle leaf could even help with skin problems. Her little cousin, Benny, had a nasty rash. Lily used nettle leaves to make a soothing salve, and Benny's skin healed faster than ever.

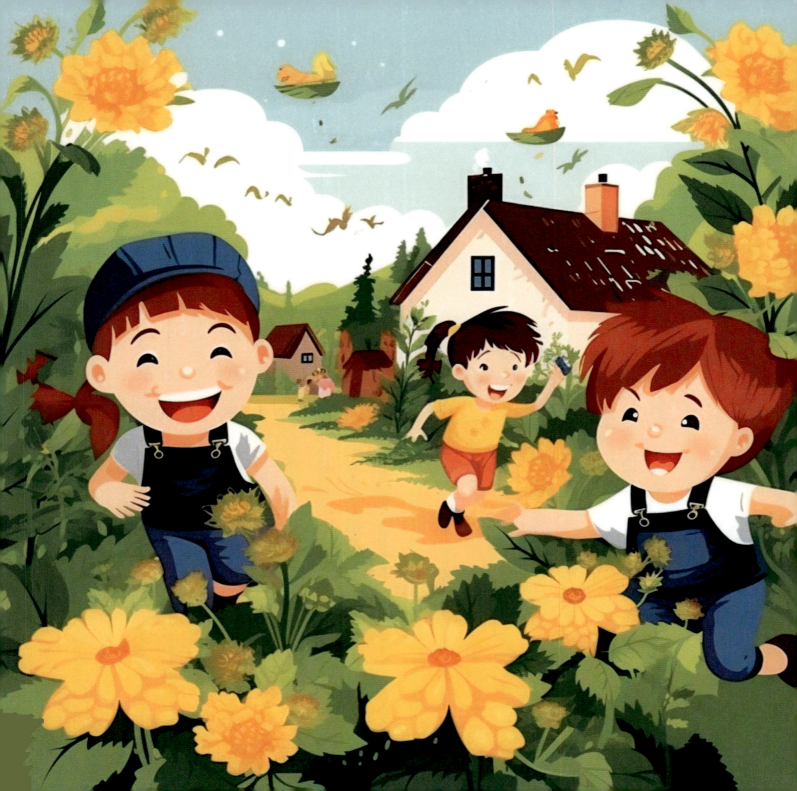

As Lily helped more friends and family with nettle leaf, the village started to learn about its magical powers. Everyone wanted to be like Lily, the herbalist. And so, a new generation of herbalists was inspired, thanks to the incredible adventures of Lily and her beloved nettle leaf.

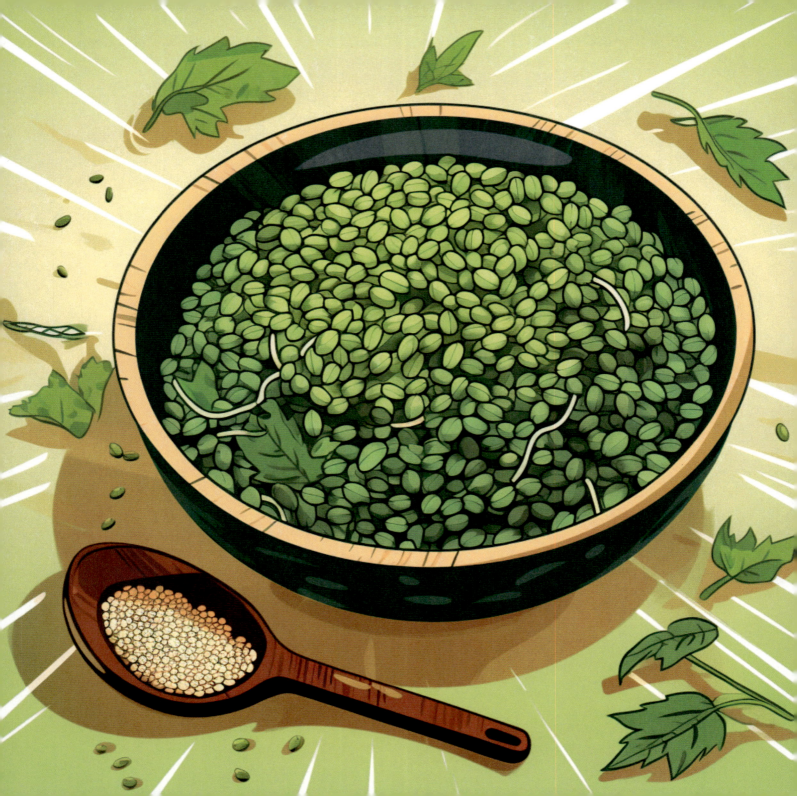

One sunny day, while Lily was exploring deeper into the forest, she came across something truly magical — nettle seeds and roots! She was overjoyed to learn that nettle had even more amazing secrets to share.

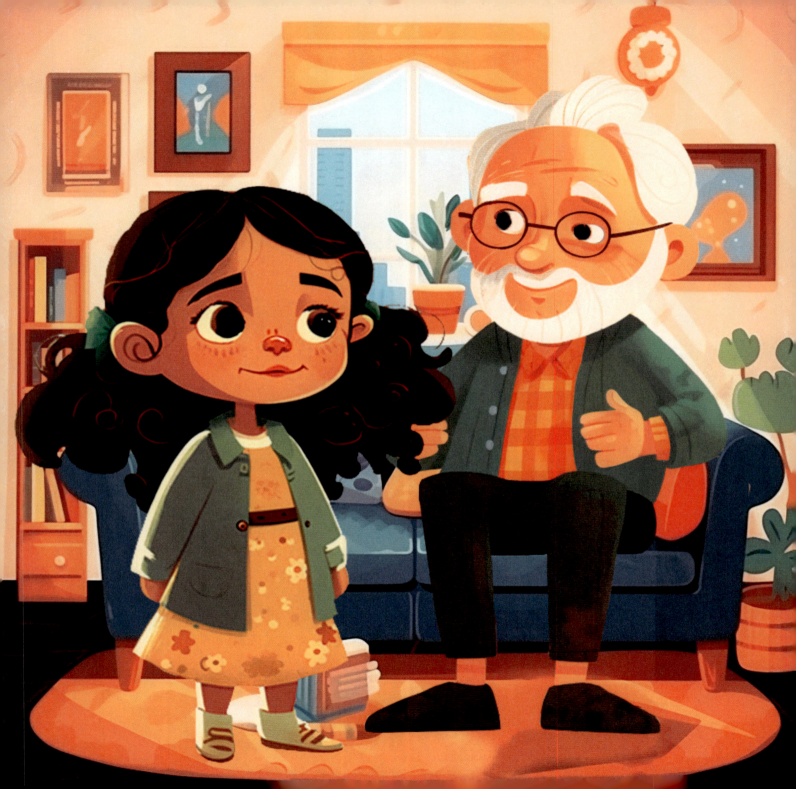

Lily discovered that nettle seeds were like tiny powerhouses. They were traditionally used as a tonic, a special kind of herb that makes everything in the body feel stronger and healthier. Nettle seeds were said to give you extra energy, just like a superhero!

Lily met her friend, Grandpa Joe, who often felt tired and worn out. She decided to share some nettle seed magic with him. She made a delicious potion with nettle seeds and gave it to him. Soon, Grandpa Joe felt more vibrant and full of life. It was as if the nettle seeds had given him superpowers!

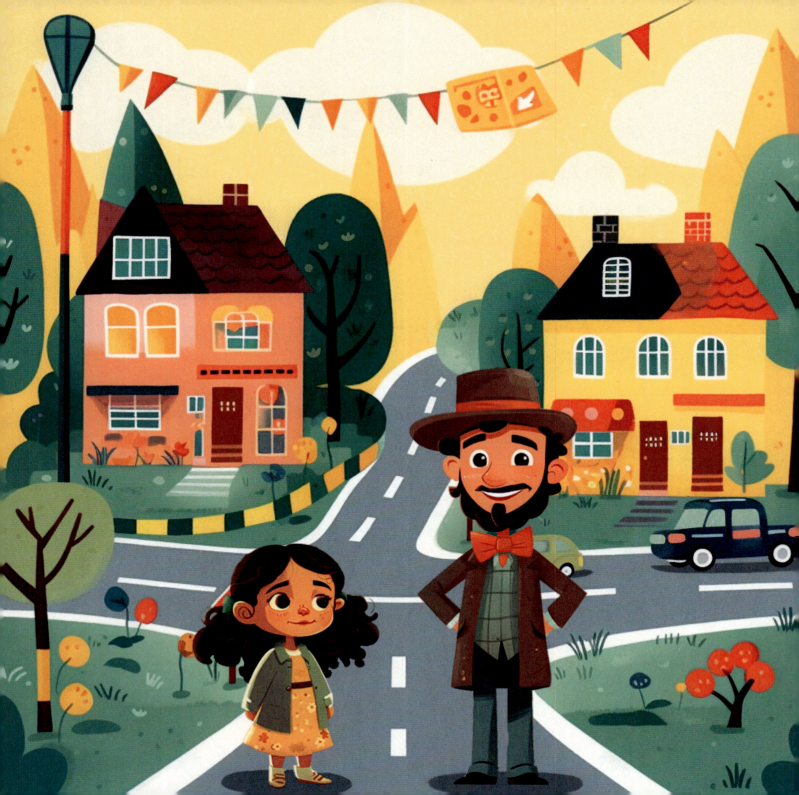

But the forest had more secrets to unveil. Lily learned about nettle roots, which had been used in herbal medicine for centuries. These roots were like nature's doctors, especially for grown-up folks.

Lily met her uncle, Mr. Smith, who had been having some trouble with his urination. He was always rushing to the bathroom, and it was causing him a lot of discomfort. Lily knew just what to do. She brewed a special tea with nettle roots and gave it to her uncle. It was like a gentle, soothing hug for his bladder.

As days went by, Mr. Smith's trips to the bathroom became less frequent, and he felt much better. Lily explained that nettle root had the power to make his prostate, a special part inside his body, feel better and not press on his bladder so much. It was like magic!

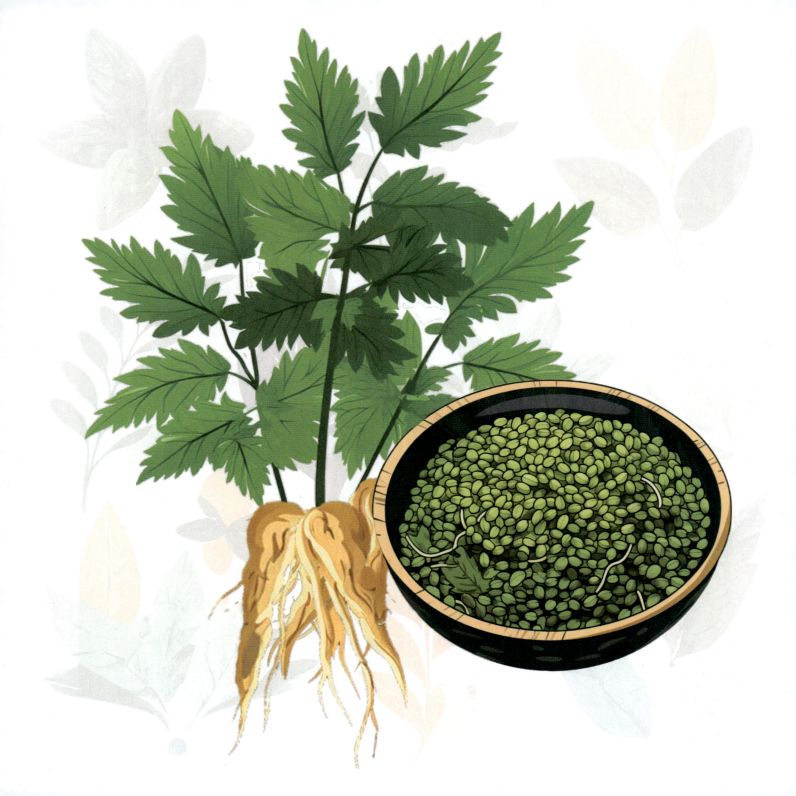

Lily was excited to share these newfound secrets with her friends and family. The village was amazed by the magical nettle seeds and roots. They were now learning that nettle wasn't just for leaves; it had incredible powers hidden in its seeds and roots too.

And so, Lily the herbalist continued her adventures, helping her village with the knowledge of nettle leaves, seeds, and roots. She had become a true guardian of nature's healing wonders, inspiring everyone to explore the world of herbal remedies.

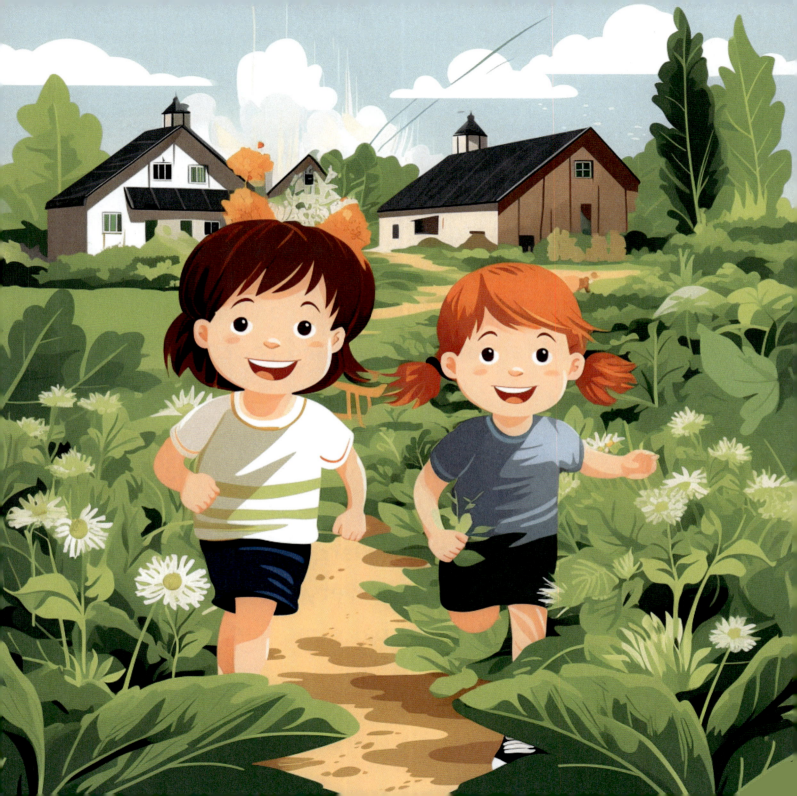

And that, my dear readers, is how Lily the herbalist and the magical nettle plant inspired a whole generation to discover the incredible world of herbal medicine. Who knows, maybe you could be the next herbalist to uncover the mysteries of nature's healing plants and help your friends and family live healthier, happier lives!

Stinging Nettle

Materia Medica

Nettle (Urtica dioica) is a versatile herb known for its various medicinal properties. It is diuretic, anti-inflammatory, nutritive, and astringent in nature. Here is a mini materia medica of nettle:

COMMON NAME: Nettle, Stinging Nettle
BOTANICAL NAME: Urtica dioica, U. urens
PARTS USED: Leaf, Seed, Root

SOME MEDICINAL PROPERTIES:

1. Diuretic: It is known for its diuretic properties, promoting the excretion of excess water from the body.

2. Anti-inflammatory: It is recognized for its anti-inflammatory properties, making it beneficial for various inflammatory conditions.

3. Nutritive: It is highly nutritious and is rich in vitamins and minerals, making it a valuable food source.

4. Astringent: It has a mild astringent quality, useful for toning and tightening tissues.

Parts and Uses

(Leaf, Seed, Root)

Nettle Leaf

Nettle leaves have been traditionally used for centuries as a nourishing and detoxifying herb. They are known for their diuretic properties, making them useful for flushing toxins from the body. It is often used to address conditions such as allergies, hay fever, and arthritis due to its anti-inflammatory properties. It may also help support urinary tract health and alleviate symptoms of benign prostatic hyperplasia (BPH) in men.

Nettle Seed

Nettle seeds are traditionally used as a tonic and rejuvenating herb. They are believed to have a strengthening effect on various body systems, including the kidneys and adrenals. They are considered an adaptogen, which means they may help the body adapt to stress and promote overall vitality. They are often used to support kidney function, boost energy, and improve resilience to stress.

Nettle Root

Nettle roots have a long history of use in traditional herbal medicine. They are primarily known for their potential benefits for the urinary and prostate health of men. It is commonly used to alleviate symptoms of BPH, such as frequent urination and urinary retention. It is believed to work by reducing the size of an enlarged prostate and improving urinary flow. Nettle root may also have anti-inflammatory effects.

Safety and Caution

CAUTION:

Nettle leaves are covered in tiny, hair-like structures that can release irritating chemicals when touched. When handling fresh Nettle (Urtica dioica) leaves wear long sleeves, gloves, and other protective clothing to minimize skin contact. Despite its notorious sting, nettle is generally regarded as a safe and beneficial medicinal plant when used appropriately. While the stinging sensation can lead to discomfort and welts, it doesn't pose significant risks when consumed as an edible or used for medicinal purposes.

PREGNANCY AND NURSING:

Pregnant and breastfeeding individuals should consult a healthcare provider before using nettle supplements.

CONSULTATION:

If you have underlying health conditions or are taking medications, consult with a healthcare professional before using nettle for medicinal purposes.

Traditional Uses

SOOTHING INJURIES:
Nettle can be used topically to soothe minor injuries such as cuts, scrapes, and bruises.

WOUNDS:
Nettle's anti-inflammatory properties help to reduce inflammation, minor wounds and promote the healing process.

BACK AND JOINT PAIN:
Nettle is often used topically to alleviate pain and inflammation associated with back and joint issues like arthritis or muscle strains.

KIDNEY AND ADRENAL ISSUES:
Nettle's diuretic and nutritive properties can be beneficial for supporting kidney function and adrenal health. It helps promote the excretion of excess water and toxins from the body.

SORE MUSCLES:
Nettle may offer relief for sore muscles.

Please note that while nettle can be helpful for these indications, it is essential to exercise caution, especially when using it topically. Always consult with a healthcare practitioner especially if you have specific medical conditions or concerns.

Recipes

Salve for Soothing Injuries, Sore Muscle and Wound Healing

INGREDIENTS:
1/2 cup Dried Nettle Leaves
1 cup Carrier Oil (e.g., Olive or coconut Oil),
2 tablespoons Beeswax

INSTRUCTIONS:
1). Fill a glass jar with the nettle leaves and pour enough carrier oil over to cover them completely.
2). Seal the jar for about 2-3 weeks, shaking it daily.
3). After the infusion period, strain the oil.
4). In a double boiler, melt beeswax and add infused oil.
5). Stir well and pour the mixture into containers. Allow it to cool and solidify. Apply topically to the affected area.

Salve for Back and Joint Pains

INGREDIENTS:
1/2 cup Dried Nettle Seed
1 cup Carrier Oil (e.g., Olive or coconut Oil),
2 tablespoons Beeswax

INSTRUCTIONS:
1). Fill a glass jar with the nettle seed and pour enough carrier oil over to cover them completely.
2). Seal the jar for about 2-3 weeks, shaking it daily.
3). After the infusion period, strain the oil.
4). In a double boiler, melt beeswax and add infused oil.
5). Stir well and pour the mixture into containers. Allow it to cool and solidify. Apply topically to the affected area.

Tincture for Kidney and Adrenal Issues

INGREDIENTS:

Nettle Seed
High-proof alcohol (e.g vodka)

INSTRUCTIONS:

1). Fill a glass jar halfway with nettle seed and pour enough high-proof alcohol over to cover them completely.

2). Seal the jar and place it in a cool, dark place for 4-6 weeks to allow tincture to develop. Shake the jar daily.

3). After the infusion period, strain the liquid and transfer into a dark (amber) glass bottle for storage.

4). Consult with a healthcare professional before using, as dosage can vary widely.

S.W.A.B.S

To remember the uses of stinging nettle for various ailments, you could use the mnemonic "SWABS"

Soothe Injuries:
Nettle Leaf + Salve

Wounds:
Nettle Leaf + Salve

Aches (Back and Joint Pain):
Nettle Seed + Salve

Bladder/Kidney and Adrenal Issues:
Nettle Seed + Tea or Tincture

Sore Muscles:
Nettle Leaf + Salve

This mnemonic encapsulates the uses of different parts of the stinging nettle plant (leaf and seed) along with the form it should be used in (salve, tea or tincture) to treat various conditions.

Thank You

Thank you for embarking on this herbal adventure with us. We hope that "Lily the Little Herbalist: Adventures with Stinging Nettle" has sparked your curiosity and passion for herbalism. May the knowledge you've gained from this book inspire your own journey as an herbalist. Happy herbal adventures!

If you're interested in further nurturing the power of imagination and herbalism, we recommend checking out these fantastic children's books:

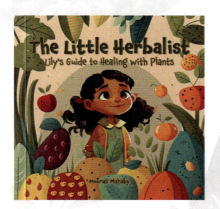 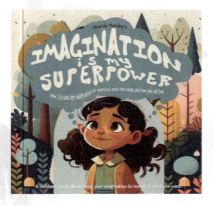 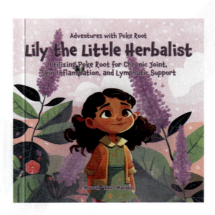

Available on www.miraherbals.info and www.amazon.com. (scan QR code)

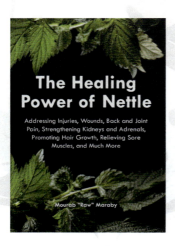

And for grown-ups seeking a deeper dive into the healing wonders of Nettle, be sure to check out, "The Healing Power of Nettle," for a wealth of knowledge on addressing injuries, wounds, back and joint pain, strengthening kidneys and adrenals, promoting hair growth, relieving sore muscles, and so much more. Start your adventure with Nettle today!

Made in the USA
Las Vegas, NV
02 April 2025

20450436R00026